Saxenda (Liraglutide) Guide:

A Step-by-Step Plan for Safe Dosing, Managing Side Effects, and Achieving Lasting Weight Loss Success.

By

Dr. Emmitt B. Leigh PhD

This publication's content is fully protected by copyright law. Reproduction, distribution, or transmission in any form or by any means, including photocopying, recording, or any electronic or mechanical methods, is strictly prohibited without prior written permission from the publisher. Short quotes may be used in reviews or for certain noncommercial purposes permitted by copyright law. Any unauthorized use or reproduction violates the copyright holder's rights.

Copyright © Dr. Emmitt B. Leigh PhD 2024.

Table of Contents

Introduction..5

Chapter 1: Understanding Saxenda...............14

Chapter 2: Starting Saxenda......................... 23

Chapter 3: Saxenda Dosing Schedule........... 33

Chapter 4: Safe Injection Techniques........... 42

Chapter 5: Managing Side Effects................ 51

Chapter 6: Lifestyle Changes for Weight Loss 62

Chapter 7: Tracking Your Progress.............. 73

Chapter 8: Dealing with Challenges............. 83

Chapter 9: Long-Term Success with Saxenda. 93

Conclusion.. 103

Introduction

Welcome to your guide on Saxenda! This book will help you understand Saxenda, why it is important for weight loss, who can use it, and what you will learn as you read through these pages.

What is Saxenda?

Saxenda is a medicine that helps people manage their weight. The active ingredient in Saxenda is called liraglutide. It comes in a pen that you use to inject the medicine under your skin. This means you put the needle into your body just a little bit, like a tiny pinch. Saxenda works by helping your body feel full, so you eat less. It can help you lose weight when combined with a healthy diet and exercise.

Saxenda is not a magic solution. It does not work by itself. You still need to make changes in your lifestyle, like eating good foods and moving your body more. Saxenda is meant for adults and children who are at least 12 years old and meet certain weight requirements.

Why is Saxenda Important for Weight Loss?

Many people struggle with their weight. Being overweight can lead to serious health problems, like heart disease, diabetes, and high blood pressure. These issues can make you feel tired and limit what you can do in life. Saxenda can be an important tool for those who need extra help in their weight loss journey.

Saxenda helps you control your appetite. When you feel full after eating, it is easier to avoid snacks and unhealthy foods. This can lead to a healthier lifestyle. When combined with good eating habits and physical activity, Saxenda can help you lose weight and keep it off for a long time.

Many studies show that Saxenda helps people lose more weight compared to just dieting alone. This means that using Saxenda can lead to better results, making it easier to reach your weight loss goals. It can also improve your overall health and help you feel better physically and mentally.

Who Can Use Saxenda?

Saxenda is approved for adults and children aged 12 years and older. However, not everyone can use Saxenda. It is important to talk to a doctor before starting this medicine.

You may be a good candidate for Saxenda if:

- You have a body mass index (BMI) of 30 or higher, which means you are considered obese.
- You have a BMI of 27 or higher and have at least one weight-related health issue, like diabetes or high blood pressure.
- You are ready to make changes in your eating and exercise habits.

Some people should not use Saxenda. This includes anyone with certain health conditions. For example, if you have a history of pancreatitis, gallbladder problems, or kidney issues, Saxenda may not be safe for you. It is essential to share your complete medical history with your doctor. They will help you decide if Saxenda is the right choice for you.

Pregnant or breastfeeding women should also avoid Saxenda, as its effects on unborn babies or breastfed infants are not fully known. Your doctor can help you find the best way to manage your weight during these important times.

What You Will Learn from This Guide

In this guide, you will find clear and simple information about using Saxenda safely and effectively. We will cover many topics to help you on your weight loss journey.

Here are some key things you will learn:

1. Understanding Saxenda: You will learn how Saxenda works, what it does in your body, and why it is effective for weight loss.

2. Starting Saxenda: We will discuss how to begin your treatment and what to expect during the first weeks of using Saxenda.

3. Dosing Schedule: You will find a step-by-step plan on how to use Saxenda

correctly, including how to increase your dose safely over time.

4. Injection Techniques: We will provide tips on how to inject Saxenda properly, so you feel comfortable and confident when using the pen.

5. Managing Side Effects: We will explain the common side effects of Saxenda and what to do if you experience any of them. Knowing how to manage side effects can make your experience smoother.

6. Lifestyle Changes: Weight loss is not just about taking medication. You will learn how to make healthy food choices and the importance of regular exercise in achieving lasting weight loss.

7. Tracking Progress: We will discuss ways to keep track of your weight loss journey, including how to celebrate small achievements along the way.

8. Dealing with Challenges: Every journey has bumps in the road. We will share strategies for overcoming challenges and staying motivated when the going gets tough.

9. Long-Term Success: Finally, we will talk about how to maintain your weight loss after stopping Saxenda. Creating healthy habits will help you enjoy a happier, healthier life.

By the end of this guide, you will have the knowledge and tools to use Saxenda effectively. You will be better prepared to manage your weight and achieve your goals.

Remember, this journey is about more than just a number on the scale. It is about feeling good, having energy, and enjoying life to the fullest. With Saxenda and the information in this guide, you can take control of your weight loss journey and make positive changes for a healthier future.

This introduction sets the stage for your book, ensuring it is clear, engaging, and informative. Let me know if you need any adjustments or additional sections!

Chapter 1: Understanding Saxenda

In this chapter, we will explore Saxenda, its main ingredient, liraglutide, how it works in your body, and why people choose to use it for weight loss. By understanding these key points, you will be better prepared to use Saxenda safely and effectively.

What is Liraglutide?

Liraglutide is a medicine that belongs to a group of drugs called GLP-1 agonists. These are long names, but they mean that liraglutide acts like a natural hormone in your body called glucagon-like peptide-1

(GLP-1). This hormone helps control your appetite and how your body handles food.

Liraglutide is used in two main ways:

1. As Saxenda for weight loss: Saxenda is the brand name for liraglutide when it is used to help people manage their weight. It is approved for adults and children aged 12 years and older who are overweight or obese.

2. As Victoza for diabetes: Victoza is another brand of liraglutide. It helps people with type 2 diabetes control their blood sugar levels.

Both Saxenda and Victoza are similar because they contain the same active ingredient, liraglutide. However, they are used for different purposes, so it is essential to use the one that your doctor prescribes.

How Does Saxenda Work?

Saxenda works in several ways to help you lose weight:

1. Feeling Full: When you inject Saxenda, it helps you feel full after eating smaller amounts of food. This is because it affects areas in your brain that control your appetite. You might notice that you don't feel as hungry as you used to.

2. Slowing Down Digestion: Saxenda also slows down how quickly food moves through your stomach. This means you will

feel full for a longer time after eating. When food takes longer to leave your stomach, it can help you eat less during meals and reduce snacking.

3. Improving Blood Sugar Levels: While Saxenda is mainly used for weight loss, it can also help improve blood sugar control. This is especially helpful for people who have diabetes or are at risk of developing it. Better blood sugar control can lead to a healthier body overall.

4. Reducing Cravings: Some people find that Saxenda helps reduce cravings for unhealthy foods. When cravings go down, it becomes easier to make better food choices. This can lead to healthier eating habits and support weight loss.

By helping you feel full, slowing digestion, and reducing cravings, Saxenda makes it easier to eat less and lose weight. It is important to remember that Saxenda is most effective when combined with a healthy diet and regular exercise.

Why Do People Use Saxenda?

Many people choose to use Saxenda for several reasons:

1. Struggling with Weight: Many individuals find it hard to lose weight through diet and exercise alone. They may have tried different weight loss programs without success. Saxenda can provide additional support for those who are determined to reach their weight loss goals.

2. Health Concerns: Being overweight can lead to various health problems, including heart disease, diabetes, and high blood pressure. By using Saxenda, people hope to reduce their weight and lower their risk of these serious health issues. Losing weight can improve overall health, making everyday activities easier and more enjoyable.

3. Long-Term Results: People using Saxenda often seek long-term weight loss results. They want to lose weight not just for a short time but to keep it off for good. Studies show that many people using Saxenda lose more weight than those trying to lose weight without medication. This can make a big difference in their lives and

motivate them to continue their healthy habits.

4. Support from Health Professionals: When people decide to use Saxenda, they usually do so under the guidance of a healthcare provider. This support can be vital in ensuring that the medication is used safely and effectively. Health professionals can help people set realistic goals, create a healthy eating plan, and encourage regular exercise.

5. Improved Quality of Life: Many individuals notice an improved quality of life after starting Saxenda. They may feel more energetic, happier, and more confident. This can lead to better relationships and a more fulfilling life.

In summary, Saxenda is a medication that helps people manage their weight by controlling appetite, slowing digestion, and reducing cravings. Liraglutide, the active ingredient, plays a crucial role in these effects. People choose Saxenda for various reasons, including struggling with weight, health concerns, and the desire for long-term results. With support from healthcare providers and a commitment to a healthier lifestyle, many individuals can achieve their weight loss goals and improve their quality of life.

As we move forward in this guide, we will cover more about how to use Saxenda safely, manage any side effects, and make lasting changes to your lifestyle. Understanding

Saxenda and its effects is the first step toward a healthier and happier you.

If you have any questions or need more information, don't hesitate to ask your healthcare provider. They are there to help you every step of the way.

Chapter 2: Starting Saxenda

Starting Saxenda is an important step in your journey to lose weight. In this chapter, we will discuss how to begin your treatment, the first steps to take, and why talking to your doctor is essential. By understanding these points, you can start Saxenda safely and effectively.

How to Begin Your Treatment

Before you start taking Saxenda, it is crucial to prepare yourself. Here are the steps to help you begin your treatment:

1. Get a Prescription: Saxenda is a prescription medication. This means you

need to get it from a doctor. Make an appointment with your healthcare provider to discuss your weight loss goals. Your doctor will assess your health, talk about your history with weight loss, and determine if Saxenda is right for you.

2. Learn About Saxenda: It's important to understand what Saxenda is and how it works. Your doctor will explain how it can help you lose weight and what you can expect while using it. This includes information about dosage, administration, and potential side effects.

3. Follow the Dosage Plan: Your doctor will provide you with a dosage plan. Saxenda is usually started at a low dose and then increased gradually. This helps your body

adjust to the medication. Following your doctor's instructions is very important to ensure your safety and effectiveness.

4. Prepare for Injection: Saxenda comes in a prefilled pen that you use to inject the medication. Before starting, you should learn how to use the pen. Your doctor or pharmacist can show you how to do this. It's essential to understand how to inject Saxenda correctly to avoid mistakes.

5. Choose the Right Time: You will need to inject Saxenda once a day. You can choose a time that fits best into your daily routine. Some people prefer to take it in the morning, while others like to take it in the evening. What matters most is that you take it at the same time every day. This helps

keep your medication levels steady in your body.

First Steps to Take

Once you have your prescription and are ready to start Saxenda, here are some important first steps to take:

1. Set Weight Loss Goals: Think about what you want to achieve with Saxenda. Setting realistic weight loss goals can help you stay motivated. It is often recommended to aim for a weight loss of about 5-10% of your total body weight in the first six months. For example, if you weigh 200 pounds, a goal of losing 10-20 pounds is realistic.

2. Create a Healthy Eating Plan: Saxenda works best when combined with a healthy diet. Talk to your doctor or a registered dietitian about creating a meal plan. Focus on eating more fruits, vegetables, whole grains, and lean proteins. Limiting sugary foods and drinks can also help you lose weight.

3. Start Exercising: Regular physical activity is a key part of weight loss. Aim for at least 150 minutes of moderate exercise each week. This can include walking, swimming, or dancing. Find activities you enjoy so that staying active becomes fun rather than a chore.

4. Keep a Journal: Consider keeping a journal to track your food, exercise, and

feelings. Writing down what you eat and how you feel can help you identify patterns and stay accountable. You can also note any side effects you experience while using Saxenda, which can be helpful for discussions with your doctor.

5. Stay Hydrated: Drinking enough water is important for your health and can help with weight loss. Aim for at least 8 cups of water each day. Staying hydrated can help you feel full and may reduce cravings for unhealthy snacks.

The Importance of Talking to Your Doctor

Communication with your doctor is key to your success with Saxenda. Here are some reasons why talking to your doctor is essential:

1. Monitoring Your Progress: Your doctor will want to check on your progress while using Saxenda. Regular appointments allow them to see how well you are doing and if any adjustments need to be made to your treatment plan. They can help you stay on track with your weight loss goals.

2. Managing Side Effects: Some people may experience side effects when starting Saxenda. Common side effects include nausea, vomiting, diarrhea, and constipation. If you experience any side effects, it's essential to talk to your doctor. They can help you manage these effects and

decide if you need to change your dosage or consider alternative options.

3. Addressing Concerns: If you have any questions or concerns about using Saxenda, don't hesitate to ask your doctor. They are there to help you understand the medication and ensure you are using it safely. Discussing your feelings and experiences can help you feel more confident in your weight loss journey.

4. Adjusting Your Plan: Your healthcare provider can help adjust your diet and exercise plan based on your progress. If something isn't working, they can suggest changes to help you stay motivated and successful.

5. Understanding Your Health: It's important to share your complete health history with your doctor. This includes any medications you are currently taking, allergies, and other medical conditions. Knowing your health background allows your doctor to provide the best care possible.

In conclusion, starting Saxenda involves several important steps. You must get a prescription, learn about the medication, and follow your doctor's dosage plan. Setting realistic weight loss goals, creating a healthy eating plan, and exercising regularly will help you succeed. Communicating with your doctor is essential for monitoring your progress, managing side effects, and adjusting your plan as needed.

By taking these steps, you can start your journey with Saxenda confidently. Remember, it is a team effort, and your healthcare provider is there to support you along the way. With the right plan and determination, you can achieve your weight loss goals and improve your overall health.

Chapter 3: Saxenda Dosing Schedule

In this chapter, we will discuss the Saxenda dosing schedule. This includes understanding what dose titration is, how to follow the dosing plan, and what to know about dosage increases. It's essential to follow the correct dosing schedule to ensure Saxenda works well for you.

What is Dose Titration?

Dose titration is a way to adjust the amount of medicine you take. For Saxenda, it means starting with a small dose and slowly increasing it. This approach helps your body get used to the medication. Here's why dose titration is important:

1. Reducing Side Effects: Starting with a low dose can help lessen the chances of experiencing side effects. Many people feel nausea or upset stomach when they first start taking Saxenda. By starting slow, your body can adjust to the medication better.

2. Finding the Right Dose: Everyone's body is different. What works for one person may not work for another. Dose titration allows your doctor to find the best dose for you. They will monitor how you feel and make changes if necessary.

3. Improving Effectiveness: Gradually increasing the dose can help make Saxenda

more effective. When your body gets used to the medication, it can work better for weight loss.

4. Staying Safe: Dose titration is a safe way to start a new medication. It helps prevent problems that can occur if you take too much medicine right away.

How to Follow the Dosing Plan

Following the dosing plan for Saxenda is very important. Here are steps to help you follow the plan correctly:

1. Start with the Initial Dose: When you begin Saxenda, you will start with a low dose. This is usually 0.6 mg per day. You will use the prefilled pen to inject the

medication. Your doctor will show you how to do this.

2. Increase the Dose Weekly: After one week, you will increase the dose to 1.2 mg. If you feel good and do not have any major side effects, you will continue to increase the dose each week. Here's the usual schedule:
  - Week 1: 0.6 mg
  - Week 2: 1.2 mg
  - Week 3: 1.8 mg
  - Week 4: 2.4 mg
  - Week 5 and beyond: 3.0 mg (this is the highest dose)

3. Keep a Schedule: It's helpful to keep a schedule for your doses. Write down which dose you take each day. This can help you

remember when to increase your dose and ensure you do not miss any injections.

4. Monitor Your Body: Pay attention to how your body feels after each dose. If you experience side effects, take notes. This information is important for your doctor. If you feel too sick or uncomfortable, let your doctor know. They might suggest waiting longer before increasing the dose.

5. Stay Consistent: Take your Saxenda injection at the same time every day. Consistency helps your body get used to the medication. It also makes it easier to remember to take it.

Understanding the Dosage Increases

As you follow the dosing plan, it's important to understand the dosage increases. Here's what you need to know:

1. Purpose of Increases: The goal of increasing the dose is to find the amount that works best for you. The final dose can help you achieve better weight loss results. However, the increases should be done carefully and slowly.

2. Possible Side Effects: When you increase the dose, you might notice side effects. Common side effects include nausea, diarrhea, and upset stomach. These effects may happen more when you first start the medication or when you increase the dose. If

you feel too uncomfortable, talk to your doctor. They may suggest adjusting the dosing plan.

3. When to Stop Increasing: If you reach the highest dose of 3.0 mg and still do not see results, or if you have ongoing side effects, your doctor may advise stopping Saxenda. It's important to communicate with your healthcare provider about how you are feeling.

4. Your Doctor's Guidance: Always follow your doctor's advice regarding dosage increases. They know your health history and can make the best decisions for your treatment. If you are uncertain about the dosing plan, ask questions. Your doctor is there to help you.

5. Adjusting the Schedule: Sometimes, your doctor may recommend a different schedule for increasing the dose based on your unique situation. It's important to be flexible and open to adjustments. Your healthcare provider will guide you in making the best choices for your weight loss journey.

Conclusion

Understanding the Saxenda dosing schedule is an essential part of starting your weight loss journey. By knowing what dose titration is and how to follow the dosing plan, you can use Saxenda safely and effectively. Remember to monitor how you feel, stay consistent with your injections, and always communicate with your doctor.

With the right approach, Saxenda can be a valuable tool in achieving your weight loss goals. Following the dosing plan can help ensure that you get the best results while minimizing side effects. Your health is a priority, so take the time to understand the dosing schedule and follow it carefully. This way, you can set yourself up for success as you work towards a healthier you.

Chapter 4: Safe Injection Techniques

Using Saxenda requires you to give yourself an injection. This chapter will guide you on how to inject Saxenda safely and comfortably. We will discuss where to inject, how to prepare for the injection, and tips for making it as pain-free as possible.

Where to Inject Saxenda

Knowing where to inject is important for both safety and comfort. You have several options for where to give yourself the injection:

1. Abdomen: The belly area is a great spot. You can inject anywhere in the stomach, but avoid the area around your navel (belly button). Make sure to stay at least two inches away from it. This area has lots of fat, which helps the medicine absorb well.

2. Thigh: You can also use the outer part of your thigh for the injection. This area is easy to reach and can be comfortable. Make sure to choose the top part of your thigh, about halfway down.

3. Upper Arm: The back of your upper arm is another good place. You might need someone to help you with this spot, as it can be hard to reach.

4. Rotation of Injection Sites: It is important to change the injection site each time you inject Saxenda. Using the same spot repeatedly can cause irritation or lumps. Rotate between different areas of your abdomen, thigh, and upper arm.

5. Check for Skin Conditions: Before injecting, look at the skin where you plan to inject. Make sure there are no cuts, bruises, or infections. If you see anything unusual, choose another site.

How to Prepare the Injection

Preparing for the injection is a simple process. Here's how to do it step-by-step:

1. Wash Your Hands: Before anything else, wash your hands thoroughly with soap and water. Clean hands help prevent germs from getting into your body.

2. Gather Your Supplies: You will need your Saxenda pen, alcohol swabs, and a sharps container for used needles. Make sure everything is within reach before you start.

3. Remove the Cap: Take off the cap from the Saxenda pen. Check the medicine in the pen to make sure it looks clear and free of particles. If you notice anything unusual, do not use the pen.

4. Attach the Needle: If your pen does not have a needle attached, take a new needle and screw it onto the pen. Be careful not to

touch the sharp part of the needle. This keeps it clean.

5. Prime the Pen: To make sure the pen works properly, you need to prime it. To do this, turn the dose selector to 0.6 mg and press the injection button. You should see a drop of medicine at the needle tip. If you don't see a drop, repeat this step until you do.

6. Clean the Injection Site: Take an alcohol swab and clean the area where you plan to inject. Allow the skin to dry. This helps prevent infection and makes the injection easier.

7. Get Ready to Inject: Hold the pen like a pencil with one hand. With your other hand,

pinch the skin around the injection site to create a small fold. This helps the needle go in more easily.

Tips for a Pain-Free Injection

Injecting Saxenda doesn't have to be painful. Here are some tips to help make your injection as comfortable as possible:

1. Relax: It is important to stay calm and relaxed. If you are tense, it may hurt more. Take a few deep breaths to help you relax before injecting.

2. Inject Quickly: When you are ready, insert the needle quickly into the skin. A quick injection can feel less painful than a slow one. Don't hesitate; just do it!

3. Angle of Injection: Insert the needle at a 90-degree angle for most injection sites. This means the needle should be straight up and down. If you are injecting into a fatty area, you might inject at a 45-degree angle, but this is usually not necessary for Saxenda.

4. Press the Button Firmly: Press the injection button firmly to deliver the medicine. Keep the needle in for a few seconds after injecting to make sure all the medicine goes in.

5. Remove the Needle: Once you've injected the full dose, pull the needle out quickly. Use a gentle motion; there's no need to yank it out.

6. Dispose of the Needle Safely: After the injection, place the used needle in a sharps container. Never throw it in the regular trash. This helps keep you and others safe from needle injuries.

7. Apply Pressure: If you notice any bleeding after the injection, gently press the area with a cotton ball or gauze. You can also apply a small bandage if needed.

8. Use a Distraction: If you are nervous about the injection, try to distract yourself. You can look at your phone, listen to music, or chat with someone while you prepare and inject.

Conclusion

Injecting Saxenda can feel intimidating, but it doesn't have to be. Knowing where to inject, how to prepare, and following tips for a pain-free injection can help make the process easier. Practice safe injection techniques to ensure that you use Saxenda effectively and comfortably.

Remember to rotate your injection sites, keep everything clean, and talk to your doctor if you have any concerns. With a little practice, you will feel more confident giving yourself the injection and staying on track with your weight loss journey. Your health is important, and following these safe injection techniques will help you use Saxenda successfully.

Chapter 5: Managing Side Effects

Using Saxenda can help many people lose weight and improve their health. However, just like any medicine, Saxenda can cause side effects. This chapter will explain the common side effects of Saxenda, what you can do if you feel unwell, and when it's important to contact your doctor.

Common Side Effects of Saxenda

When you start using Saxenda, you may notice some side effects. Not everyone will experience these, and many side effects are mild. Here are some common side effects you might encounter:

1. Nausea: This is when you feel like you might throw up. It's one of the most common side effects. Nausea usually happens when you first start taking Saxenda. It might go away after a few days or weeks as your body gets used to the medicine.

2. Vomiting: Sometimes, nausea can lead to vomiting. If you feel very sick, you might throw up. If this happens, drink clear fluids to stay hydrated.

3. Diarrhea: This is when you have loose or watery stools. Diarrhea can make you feel uncomfortable, but it often gets better on its own. Make sure to drink plenty of water so you don't get dehydrated.

4. Constipation: This is when you have trouble going to the bathroom or have hard stools. Eating more fiber and drinking water can help prevent constipation.

5. Stomach Pain: You might feel pain or cramps in your belly. This can happen when your body is adjusting to Saxenda. If the pain is severe or doesn't go away, talk to your doctor.

6. Loss of Appetite: Some people may not feel as hungry when taking Saxenda. This can be helpful for weight loss, but make sure to eat enough healthy food.

7. Headaches: You might experience headaches, especially when you first start

the medication. Drinking water and resting can help reduce headaches.

8. Fatigue: Some users report feeling more tired than usual. Make sure to get enough sleep and rest when needed.

9. Dizziness: Feeling dizzy can happen, especially if you stand up quickly. If you feel dizzy, sit down until the feeling passes.

10. Changes in Heart Rate: Saxenda can affect your heart rate. You might notice your heart beating faster or slower than usual.

Most of these side effects are temporary and will go away as your body gets used to the medication. It is important to keep track of how you feel and what side effects you notice.

What to Do If You Feel Unwell

If you experience any side effects, here are some steps you can take to help yourself feel better:

1. Stay Hydrated: If you feel nauseous or have diarrhea, it is very important to drink plenty of fluids. Water is best. You can also try clear broth or electrolyte drinks to keep your body balanced.

2. Eat Small Meals: If you have a poor appetite or feel nauseous, try eating small meals throughout the day instead of three

large meals. Eating smaller amounts can help reduce nausea.

3. Rest: If you feel tired or fatigued, allow yourself to rest. Take breaks and do activities that are calming and gentle.

4. Manage Pain: If you have stomach pain or headaches, over-the-counter pain relievers like acetaminophen or ibuprofen can help. However, always check with your doctor before taking any new medication.

5. Keep a Diary: Write down the side effects you experience, including when they happen and how severe they are. This can help you and your doctor understand your body's reactions better.

6. Talk to Friends or Family: Sharing how you feel with someone you trust can help. They might have tips or can support you during this time.

When to Contact Your Doctor

While most side effects are mild and temporary, there are some situations when you should contact your doctor right away. Here are signs that mean you should get help:

1. Severe Nausea or Vomiting: If nausea or vomiting becomes very intense and does not go away, contact your doctor. You may need medication to help with this.

2. Severe Stomach Pain: If you experience strong pain in your abdomen that doesn't get better, it's important to reach out to your doctor. They may want to check for any serious issues.

3. Dehydration: Signs of dehydration include extreme thirst, dry mouth, very dark urine, or feeling dizzy when standing up. If you notice these symptoms, call your doctor.

4. Allergic Reactions: If you develop a rash, itching, swelling of your face, lips, or tongue, or have difficulty breathing, seek immediate medical help. These could be signs of a serious allergic reaction.

5. Changes in Mood or Behavior: If you notice significant changes in your mood,

such as feeling very sad or anxious, let your doctor know. Sometimes, medications can affect how we feel.

6. Heart Rate Changes: If you feel your heart racing or pounding in an unusual way, especially if you feel dizzy or lightheaded, contact your doctor. This can help ensure your heart is healthy.

7. Unusual Fatigue: If you feel extreme tiredness that interferes with your daily activities, it's important to talk to your doctor. They may need to assess your overall health.

8. Persistent Side Effects: If any side effect lasts longer than a few days or worsens, call

your doctor for advice. They may need to adjust your dosage or provide support.

Conclusion

Managing side effects is an important part of using Saxenda. Knowing what to expect can help you feel more prepared. Remember that many side effects are common and often go away as your body adjusts. Staying hydrated, eating small meals, and resting can help ease discomfort.

Always pay attention to how you feel and don't hesitate to reach out to your doctor if something doesn't feel right. Your health and safety are very important. By managing side effects carefully, you can stay on track with your weight loss journey and enjoy the benefits that Saxenda has to offer.

Chapter 6: Lifestyle Changes for Weight Loss

Using Saxenda can help you lose weight, but it works best when you also make healthy lifestyle changes. This chapter will explain how to eat healthy while using Saxenda, the importance of exercise, and tips on how to stay motivated on your weight loss journey.

Eating Healthy While Using Saxenda

Eating healthy is an important part of losing weight. Saxenda helps you feel less hungry, but you still need to choose the right foods. Here are some tips to help you eat healthier:

1. Focus on Fruits and Vegetables: Fruits and vegetables are full of vitamins, minerals, and fiber. They can help you feel full without adding too many calories. Try to fill half your plate with colorful fruits and vegetables at every meal.

2. Choose Whole Grains: Whole grains, like brown rice, whole wheat bread, and oatmeal, are better than white grains. They have more nutrients and fiber, which can help you feel satisfied for longer.

3. Include Lean Proteins: Foods like chicken, fish, beans, and nuts are great sources of protein. Protein helps build muscles and keeps you feeling full. Try to include a source of lean protein in every meal.

4. Watch Portion Sizes: Even healthy foods can lead to weight gain if you eat too much. Use smaller plates to help control your portions. Remember, it's okay to leave food on your plate if you feel full.

5. Limit Sugary and Processed Foods: Foods like candy, soda, and fast food are often high in sugar and unhealthy fats. These foods can add a lot of calories without making you feel full. Try to limit these foods and choose healthier snacks like fruits or nuts instead.

6. Stay Hydrated: Drinking enough water is very important. Sometimes, when you feel hungry, you may just be thirsty. Aim for at least 8 glasses of water a day. Herbal teas and water with lemon can also be refreshing options.

7. Plan Your Meals: Planning your meals in advance can help you make healthier choices. Take time each week to decide what you will eat. This can prevent last-minute decisions that might not be healthy.

8. Keep a Food Diary: Writing down what you eat can help you stay aware of your choices. A food diary can also help you see patterns in your eating habits. You might notice times when you eat out of boredom or stress.

By focusing on healthy eating, you can maximize the benefits of Saxenda and support your weight loss goals.

The Role of Exercise

Exercise is another important part of losing weight. It helps you burn calories, builds muscle, and keeps your heart healthy. Here are some tips on how to include exercise in your routine:

1. Start Slow: If you are not used to exercising, start with small activities. Walking for 10 to 15 minutes a day is a great way to begin. As you get more comfortable, gradually increase the time and intensity of your workouts.

2. Find Activities You Enjoy: Exercise doesn't have to be boring. Try different activities to find what you like. You might enjoy dancing, swimming, biking, or playing

sports. The more you enjoy it, the more likely you are to stick with it.

3. Set Realistic Goals: Set small, achievable goals for your exercise routine. For example, you might aim to walk for 30 minutes a day, five days a week. When you reach your goal, reward yourself with something fun, like a movie night or new workout gear.

4. Mix It Up: Doing a variety of exercises can help you work different muscles and prevent boredom. Try to include a mix of aerobic activities (like running or cycling) and strength training (like lifting weights or doing yoga) in your routine.

5. Stay Active Throughout the Day: Look for ways to be active during your day. Take the

stairs instead of the elevator, walk or bike to nearby places, or do some stretches while watching TV. Every little bit counts!

6. Make Exercise a Habit: Try to set aside a specific time each day for exercise. It can help to treat it like an important appointment. Consistency is key to making exercise a regular part of your life.

7. Listen to Your Body: It's important to pay attention to how your body feels during exercise. If you feel pain or discomfort, stop and rest. It's okay to take breaks or modify exercises to suit your comfort level.

8. Join a Group or Class: Sometimes exercising with others can keep you motivated. Look for local classes, clubs, or

groups where you can meet people who are also interested in fitness.

By making exercise a regular part of your life, you can boost your weight loss efforts and improve your overall health.

How to Stay Motivated

Staying motivated can be challenging, but it is very important for long-term success. Here are some tips to help you stay on track:

1. Set Clear Goals: Write down specific goals for your weight loss journey. For example, aim to lose a certain amount of weight or fit into a specific clothing size. Make sure your goals are realistic and achievable.

2. Track Your Progress: Keep a journal or use an app to track your food intake, exercise, and weight loss. Seeing your progress can be very encouraging. Celebrate each small success along the way.

3. Reward Yourself: Set up a system of rewards for when you reach your goals. Treat yourself to something special, like a new book, a spa day, or a fun outing. Just make sure your rewards are not food-related!

4. Stay Positive: Surround yourself with positive influences. Spend time with friends and family who support your goals. Avoid negative talk about weight or body image.

5. Visualize Your Success: Imagine how you will feel and look once you reach your weight loss goals. Picture yourself enjoying activities you love, like playing with your kids or fitting into your favorite clothes.

6. Be Kind to Yourself: Remember that setbacks can happen. If you have a bad day or week, don't be too hard on yourself. Learn from it and get back on track. It's a journey, and it's okay to have ups and downs.

7. Stay Educated: Learn more about healthy eating and exercise. The more you know, the more empowered you will feel. Read books, watch videos, or follow experts on social media for inspiration.

8. Connect with Others: Consider joining a support group or online community where you can share your experiences and challenges. Connecting with others who have similar goals can provide encouragement and motivation.

Making healthy lifestyle changes takes time and effort, but it is worth it. By focusing on good eating habits, regular exercise, and staying motivated, you can achieve lasting weight loss success with the help of Saxenda. Remember, you are not alone on this journey, and every step you take brings you closer to your goals.

Chapter 7: Tracking Your Progress

Tracking your progress is a key part of losing weight and staying healthy. It helps you see how far you've come and what changes you need to make. In this chapter, we will talk about why tracking is important, how to keep a food and weight journal, and how to celebrate your small wins.

Why Tracking is Important

Tracking helps you understand your habits and progress. Here are a few reasons why it is important:

1. Awareness: When you write down what you eat and how much you weigh, you become more aware of your choices. This awareness can help you make better decisions.

2. Accountability: Keeping track of your progress holds you accountable. You are more likely to stick to your goals if you see them written down.

3. Identifying Patterns: By tracking your food and weight, you can see patterns in your eating and activity. For example, you might notice that you eat more when you are stressed or that you tend to skip meals.

4. Measuring Success: Tracking allows you to measure your success. You can see how

much weight you've lost or how your eating habits have improved over time. This can motivate you to keep going.

5. Adjusting Your Plan: If you find that you are not making progress, tracking can help you figure out why. You may need to adjust your eating habits or exercise routine.

Overall, tracking is a useful tool that helps you stay on the right path toward your weight loss goals.

How to Keep a Food and Weight Journal

Keeping a food and weight journal is simple and effective. Here's how to do it:

1. Choose Your Journal: You can use a notebook, a planner, or a smartphone app to

track your progress. Find a method that works best for you.

2. Record Your Food: Every time you eat, write down what you had. Be specific about the food and portion size. For example, instead of writing "salad," you can write "1 cup of mixed greens with 2 tablespoons of dressing."

3. Note the Time: Write down the time you eat each meal or snack. This can help you see if you are eating at regular times or if you are snacking too much.

4. Track Your Feelings: Along with food, write down how you feel before and after eating. Are you hungry, bored, or stressed?

This can help you understand your eating triggers.

5. Weigh Yourself Regularly: Choose a specific day each week to weigh yourself. Write down your weight in your journal. It's best to weigh yourself at the same time each week, like in the morning after you wake up.

6. Reflect on Your Progress: At the end of each week, take some time to review what you've written. Look for patterns in your eating habits, weight changes, and feelings. This can help you see what is working and what needs to change.

7. Be Honest: It's important to be honest in your journal. Don't skip over the foods that are not healthy or the days when you didn't

stick to your plan. This honesty will help you improve.

8. Stay Consistent: Make tracking a daily habit. The more consistent you are, the more helpful your journal will be.

Keeping a food and weight journal is a powerful way to stay focused on your goals and make positive changes.

Celebrating Small Wins

Celebrating small wins is important for staying motivated. Here are some ideas on how to recognize and celebrate your achievements:

1. Set Small Goals: Break your big goals into smaller, achievable steps. For example, instead of aiming to lose 30 pounds, set a goal to lose 5 pounds first. Celebrate when you reach that first goal!

2. Reward Yourself: Choose non-food rewards to celebrate your wins. This could be a movie night, new workout clothes, or a fun day out. Rewards can help keep you excited about your progress.

3. Share Your Success: Tell friends and family about your achievements. Sharing your success can make it even more special. They might celebrate with you or offer support for your next goal.

4. Take Photos: Document your progress with photos. Take pictures of yourself at different stages of your weight loss journey. Seeing how you change over time can boost your confidence.

5. Create a Vision Board: Make a vision board with images and quotes that inspire you. Include pictures of your goals, such as healthy foods, exercise activities, and places you want to visit. Hang it where you will see it often.

6. Reflect on Your Journey: Take time to look back on how far you've come. Write down all the positive changes you've made in your eating habits, activity levels, and mindset. Recognizing your progress can help you stay motivated.

7. Keep it Fun: Find ways to make your weight loss journey enjoyable. Try new healthy recipes, join a fun exercise class, or invite a friend to work out with you. The more fun you have, the easier it will be to stay on track.

8. Stay Positive: Focus on the positive changes you've made rather than what you still need to achieve. Celebrate your hard work and dedication, no matter how small the victory.

Tracking your progress and celebrating small wins can keep you motivated and engaged in your weight loss journey. Remember that every step forward is important, and each small victory brings you closer to your ultimate goal. With

Saxenda and a commitment to healthy habits, you can achieve lasting weight loss success.

Chapter 8: Dealing with Challenges

Every journey has its bumps in the road, and losing weight is no different. It can be tough, but with the right tools and mindset, you can overcome these challenges. In this chapter, we will talk about how to deal with plateaus in weight loss, handle temptations and cravings, and find support from others.

Overcoming Plateaus in Weight Loss

A plateau happens when you stop losing weight even though you are doing everything right. This can be frustrating, but it is normal. Here are some ways to overcome plateaus:

1. Review Your Food Journal: Go back and look at what you have been eating. Are you sticking to your healthy eating plan? Sometimes we might eat a little more without realizing it. Tracking your food can help you find any sneaky calories.

2. Change Your Routine: If you have been doing the same exercises for a while, your body might get used to them. Try changing your workout. If you usually walk, try running or cycling. Mixing things up can help jumpstart your weight loss again.

3. Increase Activity Levels: Look for ways to move more during the day. This could be taking the stairs instead of the elevator, going for a walk during lunch, or doing

some gardening. Even small changes can add up.

4. Stay Hydrated: Sometimes, we confuse thirst with hunger. Make sure you are drinking enough water throughout the day. This can help you feel full and may prevent you from eating when you don't need to.

5. Get Enough Sleep: Sleep is very important for weight loss. When you don't get enough rest, your body can make more hunger hormones. Aim for 7 to 9 hours of sleep each night to help your body work its best.

6. Be Patient: Remember that weight loss is not always a straight line. It is okay to have ups and downs. Stay positive and keep

working toward your goals. With time, the scale will move again.

7. Consult with Your Doctor: If you are stuck on a plateau for a long time, talk to your doctor. They can help you find out if there is something else going on or suggest ways to get back on track.

Handling Temptations and Cravings

Temptations and cravings are a part of life. It is normal to want to eat your favorite foods, but learning how to handle these urges is key to staying on track. Here are some tips:

1. Identify Triggers: Understand what triggers your cravings. Is it stress, boredom,

or seeing your favorite food? Knowing what makes you crave certain foods can help you find ways to deal with those feelings without eating.

2. Practice Mindful Eating: When you eat, focus on your food. Take your time, enjoy each bite, and pay attention to how your body feels. This can help you feel satisfied with smaller portions.

3. Have Healthy Snacks Ready: Keep healthy snacks nearby to help curb cravings. This could be fruits, vegetables, or nuts. When you feel hungry, reaching for something healthy can keep you from going for unhealthy options.

4. Use the 10-Minute Rule: When you feel a craving, wait 10 minutes before giving in. This can help you decide if you are really hungry or if it is just a passing thought. Sometimes, the craving will go away on its own.

5. Find Alternative Activities: Instead of reaching for food when you feel tempted, find other activities to keep your mind busy. Go for a walk, read a book, or call a friend. Keeping your hands and mind occupied can help you avoid eating.

6. Allow Yourself Treats: It is okay to have your favorite foods sometimes. The key is moderation. Instead of having a whole cake, have a small slice. This way, you can enjoy what you love without feeling guilty.

7. Stay Positive: If you give in to a craving, don't be too hard on yourself. It happens to everyone. Acknowledge it, learn from it, and move on. Staying positive will help you keep your focus on your goals.

Finding Support from Others

Having support can make a big difference in your weight loss journey. Here are some ways to find support from others:

1. Share Your Goals: Talk to friends and family about your weight loss goals. Let them know how they can support you. They might join you in your healthy eating or exercise plans.

2. Join a Support Group: Look for weight loss support groups in your area or online. Being part of a group can help you feel less alone and give you motivation. You can share tips, experiences, and encouragement with each other.

3. Buddy System: Find a friend or family member who wants to lose weight too. You can work out together, share healthy recipes, and keep each other accountable. Having a buddy can make the journey more fun.

4. Seek Professional Help: If you feel you need more help, consider talking to a dietitian or a therapist. They can provide expert advice and support tailored to your needs.

5. Use Social Media: Many people share their weight loss journeys on social media. You can find inspiration and connect with others who are working toward similar goals. Just remember to focus on positive accounts that uplift you.

6. Celebrate Together: When you achieve a goal, share the moment with your supporters. Celebrating your success together can make it feel even more special and encourage everyone to keep going.

7. Be Open to Feedback: Sometimes, friends and family might have helpful advice. Be open to their suggestions and consider what works for you.

Dealing with challenges is part of the weight loss journey. By learning to overcome plateaus, handling cravings, and finding support, you can stay focused and keep moving forward. Remember that you are not alone. Many people face these challenges, and with determination and help from others, you can achieve your weight loss goals. With Saxenda and a supportive network, you are on your way to a healthier, happier life.

Chapter 9: Long-Term Success with Saxenda

Losing weight is not just about using Saxenda; it's about keeping that weight off for a long time. Many people want to enjoy their new, healthier life even after stopping the medication. In this chapter, we will talk about setting realistic goals, maintaining a healthy lifestyle after stopping Saxenda, and preparing for life after Saxenda. These steps will help you stay healthy and happy.

Setting Realistic Goals

Setting goals is important for success. When you set goals, you know what you want to achieve. However, it is very important to make sure these goals are realistic. Here's how to set goals that are easy to reach:

1. Make Specific Goals: Instead of saying, "I want to lose weight," say, "I want to lose 5 pounds in one month." Specific goals help you see exactly what you want to achieve.

2. Set Small Steps: Break your big goals into smaller steps. If you want to lose 20 pounds, you can set a goal to lose 1 pound a week. This makes your goal feel less overwhelming and helps you stay motivated.

3. Be Flexible: Sometimes things don't go as planned. If you don't reach your goal in the time you wanted, it's okay! Be flexible and adjust your goals if you need to. The important thing is to keep trying.

4. Focus on Healthy Habits: Instead of only focusing on weight loss, set goals for healthy habits. For example, aim to exercise for 30 minutes a day or eat five servings of fruits and vegetables each day. These habits will help you stay healthy, no matter what the scale says.

5. Celebrate Your Achievements: When you reach a goal, no matter how small, take time to celebrate. This could be treating yourself to a movie, a new book, or something else you enjoy. Celebrating helps you feel proud of your hard work.

6. Stay Positive: Keep a positive attitude about your goals. If you have a bad day, don't give up. Everyone has ups and downs. Focus on what you can do better tomorrow.

By setting realistic goals, you can build a path toward long-term success with your weight loss journey.

Maintaining a Healthy Lifestyle After Stopping Saxenda

Once you finish your treatment with Saxenda, it's important to keep living a healthy lifestyle. Here are some ways to maintain your healthy habits:

1. Keep Eating Healthy Foods: Continue to make good food choices. Fill your plate with fruits, vegetables, whole grains, lean proteins, and healthy fats. Eating a balanced diet will help you feel good and maintain your weight.

2. Stay Active: Exercise should still be a part of your daily life. Find activities you enjoy, like walking, dancing, swimming, or playing a sport. Aim for at least 150 minutes of exercise each week. Regular physical activity helps keep your weight steady.

3. Drink Plenty of Water: Water is important for your body. It keeps you hydrated and helps you feel full. Try to drink at least 8 cups of water a day. This can also help you avoid mistaking thirst for hunger.

4. Plan Your Meals: Meal planning can help you stick to healthy eating. Take time each week to plan what you will eat. This way, you can avoid unhealthy choices when you are busy or tired.

5. Listen to Your Body: Pay attention to how your body feels. Eat when you are hungry and stop when you are full. Learning to listen to your body can help you maintain a healthy weight.

6. Manage Stress: Stress can lead to unhealthy eating habits. Find ways to manage stress, like practicing yoga, meditating, or spending time with friends and family. Staying calm can help you make better choices.

7. Keep a Routine: Try to keep a daily routine that includes meals, exercise, and sleep. A routine can help you stay on track and make healthy choices a regular part of your life.

Maintaining a healthy lifestyle after stopping Saxenda is key to long-term success. By sticking to your healthy habits, you can continue to feel great and stay at a healthy weight.

Preparing for Life After Saxenda

As you get ready to finish your treatment with Saxenda, it's important to prepare for life after the medication. Here are some tips to help you make a smooth transition:

1. Review Your Progress: Take time to look back at your weight loss journey. What worked well? What challenges did you face? Understanding your experiences can help you plan for the future.

2. Create a Support System: Make sure you have a group of friends or family who support your healthy lifestyle. This support can help you stay motivated and accountable. You can also consider joining a support group for people who are on similar journeys.

3. Develop a Maintenance Plan: Write down a plan for how you will maintain your weight after stopping Saxenda. This could include your healthy eating habits, exercise routine, and ways to manage cravings or stress.

4. Stay Informed: Keep learning about health and nutrition. Read books, follow health blogs, or attend workshops. The more you know, the better choices you can make.

5. Check-In with Your Doctor: Schedule regular check-ups with your doctor after stopping Saxenda. They can help you monitor your weight and overall health. This is also a great time to ask any questions you might have.

6. Be Kind to Yourself: Remember that it is okay to have setbacks. If you gain a little weight back or find it hard to stay on track, be gentle with yourself. Acknowledge the challenge and refocus on your goals.

7. Set New Goals: After you finish Saxenda, think about new goals you want to achieve. This could be trying a new sport, reaching a new fitness level, or learning to cook healthy meals. Setting new goals can keep you motivated and excited.

By preparing for life after Saxenda, you can ensure that you continue to lead a healthy and fulfilling life. The skills and habits you have built during your journey will help you succeed for years to come.

In conclusion, long-term success with Saxenda is about more than just losing weight; it's about maintaining a healthy lifestyle and preparing for the future. By setting realistic goals, staying active, eating well, and seeking support, you can achieve lasting health and happiness. Remember, this journey is yours, and every step counts. Embrace your progress, and keep moving forward!

Conclusion

As we come to the end of this guide, it's important to look back at what we have learned about Saxenda and how it can help with weight loss. This journey is about more than just taking a medication. It's about creating healthy habits that can last a lifetime. In this conclusion, we will recap the key points we discussed, reflect on the journey to lasting weight loss, and offer encouragement for your success.

Recap of Key Points

Throughout this guide, we have covered many important topics related to Saxenda and weight loss:

1. What is Saxenda?: We learned that Saxenda is a medication containing liraglutide. It helps people lose weight by controlling appetite and making them feel full.

2. How to Start Saxenda: We talked about the importance of consulting your doctor before starting treatment. They can help you decide if Saxenda is right for you.

3. Dosing Schedule: We discussed how to follow the dosing schedule and the process of dose titration. It is crucial to follow your doctor's instructions to get the best results.

4. Safe Injection Techniques: We covered how to inject Saxenda safely. Knowing

where and how to inject can make the process easier and less painful.

5. Managing Side Effects: We learned about common side effects and what to do if you feel unwell. Knowing how to manage side effects can make the experience more comfortable.

6. Lifestyle Changes for Weight Loss: We discussed the importance of healthy eating and exercise. Making these lifestyle changes is key to achieving and maintaining weight loss.

7. Tracking Your Progress: We emphasized the importance of tracking your food intake and weight. Keeping a journal can help you

stay accountable and see how far you've come.

8. Dealing with Challenges: We looked at how to overcome weight loss plateaus, handle cravings, and seek support from others. Challenges are a normal part of any journey, but you can overcome them.

9. Long-Term Success with Saxenda: We talked about how to maintain a healthy lifestyle after stopping Saxenda. Setting realistic goals and having a maintenance plan are important for long-term success.

By remembering these key points, you can build a strong foundation for your weight loss journey.

The Journey to Lasting Weight Loss

The path to lasting weight loss is not always easy, but it is worth it. Each step you take brings you closer to your goals. This journey involves more than just losing weight; it's about changing your habits and creating a healthier lifestyle. Here are some important ideas to keep in mind as you move forward:

1. It's a Process: Weight loss takes time. It's important to be patient with yourself. Every small change you make adds up, so celebrate your progress, no matter how small.

2. Focus on Health, Not Just Numbers: While the scale is one way to measure progress, it's not the only way. Pay attention

to how you feel, your energy levels, and your overall health. These are just as important as the number on the scale.

3. Be Kind to Yourself: Sometimes, you may have days where things don't go as planned. That's okay! What matters is that you keep trying. Learn from setbacks and keep moving forward.

4. Create a Support System: Surround yourself with supportive people. Friends and family can encourage you, and joining a support group can help you connect with others on similar journeys. Sharing experiences makes the journey easier.

5. Stay Committed: Commitment is key to achieving your goals. Remind yourself why

you started this journey and keep your goals in mind. Staying focused will help you maintain your motivation.

6. Adapt and Adjust: Your journey may change over time. Be willing to adjust your goals and strategies as needed. What works for you now may change in the future, and that's perfectly okay.

7. Remember Your Achievements: Look back at how far you've come. Keep track of your successes, both big and small. This will help you stay motivated and remind you that you are capable of reaching your goals.

Encouragement for Your Success

As you continue on your journey to lasting weight loss, remember that you are not alone. Many people have faced the same challenges, and they have found success. You can too! Here are some encouraging thoughts to keep in mind:

- You Are Strong: You have the strength to make positive changes. Believe in yourself and your ability to succeed. Every choice you make matters.

- It's Okay to Ask for Help: If you find yourself struggling, don't hesitate to seek help. Whether it's talking to a doctor, a nutritionist, or a supportive friend, asking for help is a sign of strength.

- Visualize Your Success: Take a moment to picture yourself achieving your goals. How will you feel? What will you be doing? This vision can motivate you to keep working towards your goals.

- Take One Step at a Time: Focus on one healthy choice at a time. Trying to change everything at once can be overwhelming. Start with small steps, and gradually build on them.

- Celebrate Your Journey: Enjoy the process. Celebrate your efforts and the new habits you are forming. Life is not just about reaching the destination but enjoying the journey along the way.

In conclusion, your journey with Saxenda can lead to lasting weight loss and a healthier lifestyle. By following the steps outlined in this guide, setting realistic goals, and staying committed to your health, you can achieve great success. Remember, every step you take brings you closer to your goals. Believe in yourself, stay positive, and keep moving forward. Your success is within reach!

www.ingramcontent.com/pod-product-compliance
Lightning Source LLC
Chambersburg PA
CBHW050318230526
45471CB00005B/2241